Burnout Breakthrough:

Make the Most of Your Time,
Your Family, Your Health,
Your Career

Christopher Burton, MD

ISBN-13: 978-1-941578-07-0

Bonus Resources

Just to say "Thank You" for reading this book, I would like to give you these additional resources 100% FREE!

Go to christopherburtonmd.com/BBB

FREE RESOURCES:
3 Ways to Declutter Your Life
Effects of Exercise on Physician Stress
Goal Setting & Legacy Ladder
Outsourcing 101
Outsourcing Vendors
Writing More Efficient Soap Notes

Discover the Keys to Getting Rid of Burnout.

Overcome the things holding you back from
a better work-life balance and
a lifestyle that you really want.

Go to christopherburtonmd.com/BBB

Dedication

To my wife,
who has been my toughest critic and faithful editor throughout this
project. Because of you, this book is ten times more readable and
enjoyable. Thank you for making me sound smart.

To my children,
who are the reason I want to not only avoid burnout but also thrive in
my career. I want to spend time with you, watch you grow up, and
avoid the regrets of missing those important milestones in your lives.
You are my reason "Why"—why I write, why I teach, why I coach.

To my friends,
who have believed in me and have encouraged me on this journey. Your
feedback, suggestions, and support have helped me create a valuable tool
that will help other physicians.

To my colleagues,
who are in the trenches every day, doing your best while struggling with
burnout. It is my pleasure to share with you some tools, tips, and stories
that can help you break out of the cycle of burnout and step into a new
version of you that enjoys the career and lifestyle that you deserve.

"My legacy will be written in the hearts of
my children and the lives I made better."

—Christopher Burton, MD

Table of Contents

Introduction

Burnout is killing doctors, literally. For some, it happens suddenly, but for many more it occurs insidiously, spreading slowly like a cancer. It undermines their health, their happiness, and their careers. It ruins the lives of their family members, their patients, and those they work with regularly.

Anyone can suffer burnout. Researchers have found high rates among teachers, athletes, and lawyers. However, the burnout rate among physicians remains one of the highest across all professions.

Sadly, physician burnout is still growing in prevalence. Thirty to seventy percent of physicians across all specialties of medicine reported experiencing feelings of burnout, which has devastating and pervasive effects, not only on the physicians themselves but also on their patients, colleagues, institutions, and families. Some experts say that physician burnout is threatening the very foundation of medicine in America.

The detachment that signals the beginning of burnout can quickly lead to medical errors and subsequently to self-destructive behavior and even suicide. Because it is not addressed in medical school, most physicians do not have the tools to address burnout so it can quickly spiral down the track of self-destruction. Substance abuse, depression, divorce, and suicide occur at much higher rates among physicians than in the general population. All are a result of physicians suffering from burnout.

Multiple articles have been published on the topic. Several notable journals describe the range of problems burnout causes for physicians, their patients, and their families, as well as the staff and institutions where they work. These studies published over the last 20 years have outlined the symptoms, causes, and prevalence of burnout among physicians. More recently, the problem has begun to receive more attention from the academic community and even from the mainstream media. Despite the fact that burnout occurs at such alarming rates, this attention has not translated into real actions or solutions for the average physician.

A couple of solutions that are frequently advocated to help with burnout are the ideas of mindfulness and resilience. These terms are used by the health care system to put the blame on the victim—the burned out physicians. Don't get me wrong. There is nothing wrong with deep breathing exercises or being fully aware of your situation. But how does that help me get home on time? How does that help me get done with my charts faster? How does that improve my relationship with my spouse and children?

The answer is that mindfulness and resilience are not going to do any of those things. Maybe I'm just a practical person. Maybe my mind is too concrete to understand those abstract concepts. But I am certain there are other physicians like me. Are you one of them? Do you want real, practical solutions that you can use instead of more abstract theories?

In *Burnout Breakthrough,* I am going to show you concrete steps to take back control of your time. You will find practical actions you can take right now to start healing yourself. I will show you a way out of the stress, frustration, and guilt many physicians feel. I wrote this book for you, to break through your burnout. This book is for people who suffer from excessive stress, over-commitment, and strained relationships. It addresses some of the most challenging problems physicians face, such as daily time management and family concerns, in a high-yield manner.

I am a lifetime student of personal growth and professional development. I enjoy learning how to be more efficient and more productive. I have discovered how to communicate and connect with my colleagues, my staff, and most importantly, my family, much more effectively. I am still discovering new ways to maximize my potential and get the most out of life. I also love sharing what I have learned with others. So in addition to passing on what I have been able to teach others through writing, workshops, and mastermind sessions, I will share with you what I have done in my life and in my career as a physician to make sure I continue to enjoy practicing medicine and have the career I want to have for the long haul.

Now it is up to you. Do not be the person who misses out on opportunities in life because you take too long to decide that you want to change. Be the kind of doctor other doctors marvel about. Be the kind of person other physicians see and say, "I don't know how they do it." Be the kind of person who takes action and does so immediately.

The productivity tips, life hacks, and career tricks that you are about to read have been proven to create positive, long-lasting results for physicians just like you. All you have to do to take back control of your career and your life is to keep reading. Each chapter will give you new insight as you strive to keep the joy in your career from slipping away. Take control of your life right now. Make it productive; make it fun. Enjoy the new life you are creating.

SECTION 1:
The Pain of Burnout

CHAPTER ONE

THE PAIN OF BURNOUT

Where does burnout come from? Why does it exist? How did it become so prevalent in medicine today? As far back as 1892, Sir William Osler captured the dichotomy of being a physician when he wrote, "The practice of medicine will be very much as you make it—to one a worry, a care, a perpetual annoyance; to another, a daily job and a life of as much happiness and usefulness as can well fall to the lot of man."

His words resonate even more today. Several studies have been done showing a wide range of burnout rates among practicing physicians: 30 to 70 percent of specialists and general practitioners, 37 to 47 percent of academic faculty and 55 to 67 percent of doctors in private practice. Even for those physicians who are not classified as being burned out, medicine can still be a worry and annoyance.

The practice of medicine has changed dramatically over the last twenty years. Time demands and workloads are rising exponentially. The endless paperwork piles up faster than we can empty our inbox. Physician autonomy has become a relic of the past as everyone from politicians to employers and insurance carriers insert themselves into the patient encounter. There is also the constant scrutiny from administrators, regulators, and lawyers. The external pressures are tremendous. We end up working more hours for less money, and some of us may not even pay off our medical school debt before we retire.

We also know that many physicians become disillusioned with health care because decision-making and patient management are often in the hands of non-clinicians who have sacrificed the quality of the patient-physician relationship for numbers. Those numbers may be patient volume, revenue, or a host of other metrics. Rightfully, physicians are becoming angry that their extensive education and experience are ignored by administrators when it comes to giving real input. Yet politicians, administrators, and insurers are adept at dumping most of the risk for those decisions onto the doctors. It is a recipe for disaster!

In addition, we live in a medical culture that emphasizes perfection, denial of personal vulnerability, and delayed gratification. There is no room to talk about burnout, and not much is being done to prevent it or treat it when burnout inevitably occurs. Even those who want to tackle the problem seem at a loss for where to begin.

Numerous factors lead to burnout, and the toll they take often seems insurmountable. Each additional challenge no longer has an additive effect on stress. In fact, the effects seem to multiply. It is truly a case where the whole is greater than the sum of its parts.

Over the last ten years, physician burnout has grown at an alarming rate. One of the more commonly referenced studies asked physicians to fill out the Maslach Burnout Inventory survey (the current gold standard for measuring burnout in research) to assess whether burnout had increased between 2011 and 2014. Of those who returned the survey, nearly 10 percent of them experienced more burnout in 2014 than they had in 2011. Correspondingly, nearly 10 percent also reported a decline in work-life balance over the same period. Furthermore, substantially higher rates of burnout and decline in work-life balance were seen when the data was segmented by medical specialty.

By comparison, the American population as a whole experienced minimal changes in burnout during the same timeframe. A similar study entitled, "Physician Burnout: It Just Keeps Getting Worse," denoted a rise in burnout among all medical specialties from 2013 to 2105. Estimates now suggest that nearly one-third of primary care physicians will leave the practice of medicine due to burnout in the coming years. This will dramatically worsen the physician shortage problem.

Burnout can start even in medical school and occurs throughout training. One of the more recent studies on burnout was done with neurology residents and fellows. Nearly 1,000 participants were surveyed, with a response rate of around 38 percent. Median age was 32 years old, and respondents were roughly equally divided between males and females. The study found that 73 percent of residents and 55 percent of fellows had at least one symptom of burnout. The nearly 20-point difference between fellows and residents was strongly correlated with the residents having much higher depersonalization scores. Residents who had lower burnout risk were those who had a strong support system and better work-life balance.

The results of burnout in physicians can be devastating, too. Physicians have a divorce rate that is estimated to be 10-20 percent higher than the general population. Nearly three-quarters (73 percent) of practicing doctors would tell their children to avoid going into the profession. Physicians are much more likely to commit suicide than non-physicians. In fact, the suicide rates for female physicians are two-and-a-half to four times that of the general population. Over 400 physicians commit suicide each year, which amounts to more than one physician every single day. These few studies are the tip of the iceberg of published evidence on burnout—all of which paint a very grim picture.

There are a variety of factors that contribute to burnout, and in the next chapter, we will cover some of the biggest sources of stress in the life of the average physician. You will likely find that many of them resonate with you. We are all going through similar challenges, so it is important to know we do not face them alone.

CHAPTER TWO
CONTRIBUTORS TO BURNOUT

THE STRESS OF CLINICAL PRACTICE

A physician's career has always been stressful. Any job that deals with independent people who are hurt, sick, and scared takes a toll over time. We have tremendous responsibility but increasingly less autonomy, thus creating the ultimate high-stress environment. Even on the best days, our energy level can still be drained by the time we head home.

Regardless of our specific medical specialty, several factors are nearly universal: the strain of being on call, the politics of our local hospital or provider group, and the inevitable personality clashes with staff and colleagues. We are also expected to play many other roles that contribute to stress, including data-entry clerk and electronic health record (EHR) technician. Recent changes in the U.S. healthcare system have drastically changed how compensation is calculated, and that adds tremendous stress. The political and interpersonal strain within a department, between clinic and provider groups, and with administration take a particular toll on the physician.

MEDICAL EDUCATION

It takes nearly a decade of post-graduate training to become a physician, and during that time, we hone our strengths, skills, and characteristics in order to compete and survive. Over that time, these traits can become hard-wired and engrained in our persona. But they are a double-edged sword, a precursor to the burnout that more than half of us will experience at some point in our careers.

In medical school, the training gears you to become a workaholic. You must pass boards, and you hope to have scores near the top of your class in order to get into your first choice of residency programs. The level of competition among medical students is only intensifying as there are more graduates each year than there are residency programs to train them.

When students enter medical school, their burnout rates are similar to the general population, but those rates increase steadily as they progress through their medical education. A study comparing first-year and third-year students found that the third-year students blamed a lack of empathy, loss of professionalism and lost idealism for their depression and burnout. A 2012 national survey of medical students estimated that 37 to 44 percent experienced burnout. Fifty-eight percent screened positive for depression and nearly 10 percent struggled with suicidal ideation in the previous 12 months. Other surveys report that over 75 percent of medical students are on some type of antidepressant or anxiolytic.

The problems continue on into residency and fellowship training programs, which foster the expectation that we have to have all the answers. We are expected to be right all the time lest we incur the wrath of a more senior resident or attending. Patients also have very high expectations for their doctors, and most of us are also taught to fear the legal ramifications if we ever do make a mistake. Subconsciously we are trained to be perfectionists.

In a recent study of surgical residents, 75 percent of them were already suffering from burnout. These young doctors are just starting out in their career and are already burned out! This does not bode well for the future of health care. Those residents and their attending physicians consistently identified the same top three barriers to seeking care for burnout. Those barriers were an inability to take time off to seek treatment, avoidance, or denial of the problem, and negative stigma toward those seeking care.

Conventional medical training produces highly successful and technically-skilled physicians, but it creates dysfunction in just about every other aspect of our lives. Why do medical schools create and condone a cutthroat system of information overload and personal deprivation, thinking that is the only way to make great doctors? Why are residency programs not doing more to break down the barriers to treating burnout, especially when they know what those barriers are?

Einstein's definition of insanity is "doing the same things over and over and expecting a different result." We need to start rethinking medical education so we can break the cycle of burnout that begins even at this early stage of a physician's career. Some of these students are facing the idea of starting a new career they already hate with a $250,000 to $500,000 debt. They feel there are not many options for them other than to press forward.

Your Specialty

Across all specialties, burnout rates range from 30 to 65 percent. The 2016 *Medscape Physician Compensation Report* had some insightful findings. Front-line care physicians like emergency room, critical care, and palliative care doctors not only experience the highest rates of burnout, but they also experience the most severe symptoms. Many rated their burnout as so intense they are thinking of leaving medicine altogether. For example, palliative care physicians often experience very high levels of burnout because the majority of their patients are elderly, frail, and very vulnerable physically and emotionally, and it is difficult to achieve meaningful improvement in their conditions.

Family practitioners, internists, and general surgeons are a close second, at nearly a 50 percent burnout rate, which is still rising. Many of these primary care physicians state that they would not choose their specialty again, and some would not go into medicine at all if they could start over again. Oncologists also increasingly suffer overwhelming feelings of exhaustion, cynicism, and burnout caused by the physically and emotionally demanding role of treating seriously ill patients and their families.

No specialty is immune to burnout, but there are some were it appears especially pervasive. I would not recommend choosing a specialty based on burnout rates, but it is something medical students need to be mindful of so that they can try to lessen their risk by instituting a plan to fight burnout in their specialty of choice.

THE ROLE OF GENDER

Female physicians who are burned out are more likely to leave clinical medicine entirely, leading the exodus at twice the rate as their male colleagues. Many feel that their role as physician is competing with their roles as a mother and spouse.

Female physicians have a tendency to spend more time with patients during office visits, and they exhibit a different communication style in which they typically spend more time discussing non-medical aspects of care like education, prevention, and psychosocial aspects.

Female physicians tend to have more female patients, and these patients are more likely to have more psychosocial challenges that accompany the usual medical conditions. Male and female patients alike tend to open up more to female doctors, and male patients have a tendency to take a more demanding tone when they have a female doctor. All of these aspects can be more emotionally draining for the doctor.

My wife and I have frequent conversations about this aspect of patient care. As a urogynecologist she is compelled to educate her patients and make them feel that their concerns have been addressed in addition to managing their medical problems. Her patients love her and are grateful for this "tender loving care," as she refers to it. However, it does take a toll on her emotional energy and on her efficiency.

Physicians are certainly not rewarded financially in today's healthcare environment for spending more time with patients. In fact, this "inefficiency" is more likely to get reprimanded by the administration and sadly, even garner unsympathetic words from colleagues who work more quickly. It may seem obvious that female physicians approach medicine differently from their male colleagues, but our current system causes them to burn out even faster.

Female physicians also face added stress from their family roles. Please do not misunderstand me. I still feel bad if I am late getting home to have supper with our children, but my wife feels it even more acutely. There is something special about the maternal instinct. Aside from the internal strain of juggling roles as physician, wife, and mother, female physicians can have a lot of external pressures as well.

I am not going to dive into a social commentary here, but the fact remains that female physicians deal with issues that male physicians will probably never face. Some employers may balk at hiring a young female physician who wants to start a family because she will need to take time off for maternity leave. In two-physician families, it is often the wife who gets asked if she will cut back or quit practicing once the baby comes. Again, a social commentary about the way things should be is beyond the scope of this book, but the current "cultural norms" do add additional stress to female physicians.

Across All Ages

Younger doctors, especially those under age 35, report higher levels of burnout. Young doctors in smaller specialty fields have extremely high rates of burnout: urology (63 percent), infectious disease (61 percent), and nephrology (53 percent). Young primary care physicians are also experiencing similar levels:

Obstetricians and internists (53 percent) and pediatricians (47 percent).

As I already pointed out, burnout is seeping into medical school as well. In 2015, one-quarter of students surveyed reported they would choose a profession other than medicine if they were starting over, citing frustration with being unprepared for the business side of medicine. Specific reasons given include not having the opportunity to learn about coding, reimbursement, employment contracts, and compensation negotiations.

Burnout can be found in every corner of medicine, but the contributors above play a large, and sometimes surprising, role in the development of burnout. Many educators that I talk to do not realize that such a high percentage of medical students are burned out. Physicians and administrators alike are surprised to learn that female physicians have a suicide rate that is double or quadruple to that of the general population. We must be mindful of the signs and symptoms of burnout for ourselves and our colleagues. We will look at those next.

CHAPTER THREE

WARNING SIGNS

Burnout occurs at varying levels across the range of practice settings, specialties, and situations and at any point in a medical career. Anyone can get burned out, and most of us do at some point in our careers. Unfortunately, burnout is not always easy to diagnose. It encompasses a broad spectrum of physical, mental, and emotional consequences. Here are some of the more commonly recognized signs and symptoms:

- Physical exhaustion
- Emotional exhaustion
- Self-doubt
- Cynicism
- Depression
- Low sense of personal accomplishment
- Strained relationships
- Divorce
- Anger management difficulties
- Disruptive behavior
- General malaise
- No enthusiasm for work
- Poor work performance
- Making mistakes
- Social and emotional detachment
- Lack of compassion
- Substance abuse

Some of the symptoms on this list are quite obvious, but others are quite subtle. You may not even notice them at first. That also makes burnout hard to diagnose and quantify. Things like cynicism and sarcasm, for example, can be an early defense mechanism against an administrator who places unrealistic demands on your schedule. Strained relationships at home may seem to be about something else initially before you realize that your attitude and judgment are clouded by stress or depression.

It helps to set aside time to reflect and do a self-checkup. I recommend at least once a quarter if not every month. Ask yourself the following questions. If you answer "yes" to more than one or two of them, you are likely experiencing burnout.

1. Are there days you dread going to work?

2. Are you frustrated with the mindless bureaucracy that goes with practicing medicine today?

3. Do you feel as though you never have enough time to get everything done?

4. Are you bitter because you feel you have no control over your own life?

5. Are you missing out on important events in your loved ones' lives because you don't have the time?

6. Are you struggling with your relationships at work or home?

7. Are you physically and mentally exhausted?

8. Have you lost the fulfillment you had when you started your career?

9. Do you find yourself making mistakes or second-guessing yourself more often?

10. Are you frustrated about the career path you are on?

11. Do you frequently think that you have made the wrong decision choosing a career in medicine?

12. Are you disappointed that your career in medicine is not as rewarding as you had hoped it would be?

13. Are you afraid of losing your career, spouse or family?

If you are fortunate, you may have a family member, friend, or colleague who will let you know when you do not seem like yourself. Do not shoot the messenger when they point out that you seem distant at home or that your work seems to be slipping. Most often they speak up about what they notice because they care. Take these observations as opportunities to evaluate where you are at in your career and in your personal life. Do an honest self-assessment and address these signs and symptoms of burnout.

Many physicians ignore burnout to their own detriment. Failure to get off this path is what leads to medical errors, divorce, substance abuse, and even suicide. I do not want you to become a statistic. That is why I am writing this book. It is why I speak to physicians and administrators. It is why I began coaching my fellow physicians. Over the coming pages, I am going to share with you specific strategies to beat burnout. These methods have been tried by hundreds of other physicians just like you. Use them. Share them. You do not have to face burnout alone.

SECTION 2:
A Cure

CHAPTER FOUR

THE RESILIENCE MYTH

Burnout is a multifaceted problem which requires a multifaceted cure. However, as you may recall from the introduction to this book, I do not find methods like "resilience" and "mindfulness" to be adequate solutions to burnout. While these slogans may look good on a memo or make for a catchy presentation, they do not translate into concrete solutions for the average physician that I talk to.

According to one author, "Resilience is an emotional competence and can be considered as behavior to be acquired during training. It consists of cognitive processes that encompass at least four dimensions: self-efficacy; planning; self-control; commitment and perseverance."

So if I am burned out is it because I am not committed enough? Is the author saying I am burned out because I lack self-control?

The concept of "self-efficacy" was even less helpful. According to Wikipedia, "Self-efficacy is an individual's belief in his or her innate ability to achieve goals . . . Individuals who have high self-efficacy will exert sufficient effort that, if well executed, leads to successful outcomes, whereas those with low self-efficacy are likely to cease effort early and fail."

So based on that definition, my problem is that I am not exerting sufficient effort? If I just tried harder I would not be burned out? How does that sound to you?

As physicians, we all have demonstrated that we are more resilient than the average person or we would not have made it into medical school, mastered the intense curriculum, gotten through residency and into practice. However, although we may be resilient in one area of life, as new challenges attack our balance in life we may not have the tools or the bandwidth to adapt. We all have limits no matter how resilient we might be. So as more stressors pile on, the theory of resilience breaks down.

The problem with the idea of resilience is that it places all of the blame on the burned-out physician. I know that my burned-out colleagues are very committed, which is why they are working late and missing out on time with their families or on time to recharge. Burned out physicians are certainly trying very hard to be good doctors, good parents, and good spouses. It is absolutely not due to a lack of effort. When burned-out physicians hear that they need to be more resilient, what they really hear is that they are a failure or that they are the problem.

What about mindfulness? The dictionary defines it as "1. the quality or state of being conscious or aware of something, and 2. a mental state achieved by focusing one's awareness on the present moment, while calmly acknowledging and accepting one's feelings, thoughts, and bodily sensations, used as a therapeutic technique."

That actually sounds good. The first step to fixing a problem is to be aware of it. I also like to live in the moment and experience life fully. As Benjamin Franklin cleverly observed, "Some people die at 25 and aren't buried until 75." I certainly do not want to be one of these people. I want to enjoy all the wonderful sites, sounds, smells, and tastes that I can.

However, just being aware of your burnout does not make it go away. Those feelings and emotions of burnout are not the ones I want to dwell in or accept. Mindfulness has been shown to decrease anxiety and improve focus in some individuals, so it does have a place. It is often used in conjunction with things like yoga, reflection, and journaling. That is great. I recommend trying all of those things.

Mindfulness is not, however, enough for the physicians who are fighting to save their career or struggling to hold their marriage together. It is a tool for decreasing the acute emotions of stress, but it should not be the only tool. My biggest problem with the mindfulness movement is that it again puts all of the responsibility for burnout on the physician's shoulders. It does not take away the foundational problems in our healthcare system or offer practical solutions for addressing the challenges burned-out physicians face every day. Like resilience, mindfulness is a good theory, but it breaks down if we expect it to be the sole solution to burnout.

Going through those cognitive exercises is not enough. You must have practical solutions to decrease the stress, not just accept it. Whereas the abstract ideas around resilience often put more pressure on physicians, I prefer practical ideas and concrete solutions that empower physicians to change their lives for the better. Instead of just focusing on the uncomfortable feelings of the moment, I prefer to focus on the possibilities of a better and more fulfilling future. Being mindful of a situation is not enough. If you want to change your circumstances you must take action. In the coming chapters, I am going to share with you the specific strategies that have worked for many other physicians. You do not have to implement all of these changes at once. Pick one or two that you can start doing today that will have the biggest impact on your career or your quality of life. Begin there and take the first steps toward your burnout breakthrough.

CHAPTER FIVE

GOALS AND YOUR LEGACY

You would not start going somewhere new without some kind of directions, and you certainly would not start out without knowing where you are going. On your journey to a burnout breakthrough, you first need to create your map. I encourage you to have a pen and paper handy as you read this chapter. You are going to start by writing down your goals. What is your goal for your career? What are your lifestyle goals? What are your family goals?

This may seem like a strange place to start, but it is the best place to start for getting rid of burnout long term. Multiple studies on success prove that in order to be successful in life you need to have goals. Moreover, people who write down their goals are 80 to 90 percent more likely to achieve those goals. I want you to be successful. I want you to get rid of burnout. I want you to have the career and lifestyle you dreamed of when you started this journey into medicine.

Most of us had a very clear picture of what we wanted our career to look like when we went into medicine. We knew what kind of patients we wanted to help, what kind of lifestyle we wanted to live, and how we wanted to contribute to our communities and the world. We had a vision for our future and the legacy we wanted to create. Unfortunately, when we are burned out and dread even going to work every day, the vision of that legacy gets left behind. It is hard to break through the burnout with a career that has lost sight of its goals and a life that has forgotten its purpose.

So think back to when you first applied to medical school. What did you want your legacy to look like when you started your career? When is the last time you even thought about your legacy? Too often we get stuck in a rut, going to work and back home again, doing the same things over and over again. We forget why we went into medicine in the first place. We forget about the difference we wanted to make in the world.

As the responsibilities and accompanying stress piles up and we start getting burned out, we start going through the motions of living and working, just trying to survive. We forget about our goals and dreams. The hopes we had for our careers, our families, and ourselves take a back seat.

Simply surviving is not what most of us had in mind for our lives. We want to thrive! We want our lives to have meaning and a purpose greater than just getting through the day. We want to have an impact on the world around us and leave a legacy of caring and compassion for our patients and families. That is why I created the Legacy Ladder to help my clients reconnect with their dreams and get clear on their goals. It provides specific steps, just like rungs on a ladder, that you need to consider in order to reach your goals.

Ask yourself these legacy questions:

1. What is the legacy that I want to leave with my life?
If we begin with the big picture of what we would like to accomplish in mind, we can narrow down to the specific things

we need to change much more precisely. We can get clarity on what things are important and what things are not. Keeping the big picture in focus can help when you face the chaos of life. Remembering your purpose and why you are doing what you do is helpful to many physicians struggling with burnout.

2. What roles do I need to be successful in to make that legacy a reality?

Your role as a physician is significant, but you may also have roles as a spouse, parent, friend, or community leader that need to be considered. It is possible that these roles will compete from time to time. When your role as doctor competes with your role as a father, what are you going to choose? When someone asks you to sit on a committee or volunteer to sit on a board, simply ask yourself if that role will move you closer to your legacy goal.

3. Do my current values and beliefs align with the legacy that I desire?

Do you see yourself as a successful physician? Do you believe that you are a good parent? When we get burned out we tend to see everything in a negative light, including ourselves. If you do not believe that you deserve better than living with burnout, nothing I teach you will make it better.

Writing down your values also helps you decide which offers you will accept and which offers you will decline. I value my weekends with my family, so when I get offers to speak somewhere I am less likely to go if I have to be gone over the weekend. If you value the arts, then sitting on the board of a local theater may be more important than being on another committee at work. On the other hand, if your career goal involves achieving leadership positions within medicine, then it may be worth your time to volunteer for your specialty society or local medical association.

4. What skills do I need to acquire or develop in order to grow into my goals?

As you look at your goals, are there things you will need to learn in order to succeed? For example, if you want to become the chief medical officer at your hospital, you may need to learn leadership skills. If you want to give presentations on your area of expertise, you may need to develop your public speaking skills.

I am an author, speaker, and coach. Of those three, writing is the only one that came naturally to me. I had some innate strengths that helped me as a coach, but they needed to be developed. Speaking, however, took more time and effort, but it was important to me to improve in that area so that I can broaden my ability to reach and teach even more physicians how to live without burnout. Just because you do not have a skill yet or feel you are not perfect at it should not hold you back. Skills can be learned as long as you know which ones you need.

5. Do I have the right habits to be successful?

If someone wants to lose weight, they have to develop the habits of eating healthfully and exercising regularly. Likewise, for me to be successful at writing this book, I had to have the habit of writing something every day. Habits, like skills, can be developed. It is important to know which ones you will need to reach your goal.

6. Am I in the right environment to grow?

Many physicians I have spoken to feel that finding a new job is the answer to their burnout. While this may be the answer for some, others, unfortunately, simply take their problems with them. They are running from the pain of burnout, instead of moving toward something better. Moving toward your goals is a much more effective way to live life. That is why I encourage my clients to write out their own Legacy Ladder before making any major decisions.

The only way to have a positive impact on the world and to be a consistently positive influence on those around you is to be intentional about creating your legacy. These things do not happen by chance. If you know what you want your career to look like, if you know what you want your family life to be like, and if you know what you want your lifestyle to look like, then the only way to get there is to be intentional about climbing your legacy ladder.

We have a choice. We do not have to live with stress and burnout. We can make a change, but it requires effort on our part. Most likely, it is not something you are going to do on your own either. When you are the one stuck in the ditch, it is often hard to get yourself out. You need someone who can reach down and give you a hand. Writing this book is my way of reaching out a hand.

In the following chapter, we are going to look at some ways to optimize your personal well-being. Taking care of others requires energy. Without it, you have little left to give. We will discuss ways to recharge your energy, so you can be the best possible version of yourself.

CHAPTER SIX

TAKING CARE OF YOUR OWN WELL-BEING

PUT ON YOUR OWN OXYGEN MASK FIRST

Do you remember the last time you were on a plane? Every airline starts off the flight with a safety briefing that includes a demonstration of what to do in the case of a loss of cabin pressure. What do they say you should do? They always say to put on your own oxygen mask first. That applies to burnout as well. Each individual physician has to address his or her own well-being before they can address their patients' needs or the needs of their family.

Caring for others requires energy. Think of it just like the money in your bank account. If you do not have any energy in your account, you cannot make a withdrawal to give to someone else. You have to save up energy by doing things to take care of yourself. There are different types of energy: physical energy, mental energy, and emotional energy. The problem for most physicians is that our energy accounts are overdrawn. Most of us do not sleep well or exercise enough so we are physically drained. Our job can be so mentally demanding that we are unable to think clearly about the issues that we have to face at home. The strain of dealing with difficult administrators, colleagues, and patients leaves us emotionally exhausted, too.

So what does putting on your own oxygen mask first look like? We will look at each type of energy and ways that you can replenish your accounts.

PHYSICAL ENERGY

How often do you exercise? If you are like most physicians, then it is something that you may struggle to include in your busy schedule. But research shows that regular exercise can actually help you manage anxiety and cope with that busy schedule even better. Physical activity, whether independently or in an exercise class, has been shown to reduce the negative effects of chronic stress and make us more resilient to future stressors.

Exercise can help control the emotional and physical feelings of stress. It also works at the cellular level. Neurons get broken down and built up just like muscles. Stressing them makes them more resilient. This is how exercise forces the body and mind to adapt. Stress and recovery are a fundamental paradigm of our biology and can have surprising effects.

Studies of medical students and of general surgeons have demonstrated a significantly decreased rate of burnout among those who exercise regularly. Also well documented is decreased number of sick days used by employees who exercise regularly, with some having up to 80 percent less time missed because of illness. With so much evidence in favor of exercise, it is surprising that employers are not requiring it at the start of every day.

Sleep is also essential for battling stress. Sleep is when we recharge our bodies and allow it to recuperate from the stressors of the day. I know that there are times when sleep is not available because of being on call or having a sick child at home. I have gone through those phases of life. Waking up every few hours to feed or rock the baby then dragging yourself to work the next morning is a challenge for any new parent. It is even worse when your workdays are long and you are burning the candle at both ends. However, those days should be the exceptions instead of the rule.

MENTAL ENERGY

Sleep is essential for our mental well-being, too. We learned in medical school that we need seven to eight hours a night to function optimally. I have heard many physicians say that they do not need that much sleep. In reality, they are lying to themselves. Most of them have simply adapted to functioning on less sleep, but they are not functioning at their full potential.

Another way to save up our mental energy is by taking breaks where we do what I call mindless activities. These can be activities like reading a non-medical book, watching funny animal videos online, or simply "putzing" as my wife likes to call it. There are moments in the day when I have lost the energy to write or return phone calls. Crazy as it may sound, sometimes doing some mindless household chore like folding laundry is a nice diversion when I am mentally exhausted.

I also find doing mentally stimulating activities can be helpful when they are not related to medicine. There are many podcasts and audiobooks that you can listen to on a wide variety of subjects. What do you like to do for a hobby? Is there something you would like to learn about? Sometimes just stepping outside of your own medical specialty will give your brain a break and re-energize you for when you go back into work mode.

Artistic expression is a healthy coping mechanism as well. My wife enjoys playing the piano. I have another friend who likes to paint and two others who play the French horn. A former colleague of mine is a big foodie and enjoys experimenting with recipes. In medical school, I had a classmate who directed a gospel choir. All of these artistic expressions are great outlets for handling stress in positive and constructive ways.

EMOTIONAL ENERGY

Emotional exhaustion is one of the hallmark signs of burnout. Unlike exercise though, which you can objectively measure in minutes a day, miles run, or reps lifted, emotional energy exertion is harder to quantify. Every interaction you have with a patient, staff member, spouse, or child requires some kind of emotional energy. The amount is not the same for every encounter, but each one makes some withdrawal from your energy account.

"Daddy, I need you." At age two, my daughter began using this phrase quite frequently. While it was cute at first, I soon realized that she was using these four words to motivate me into doing her wishes. She had already learned that if she needed me, I would be there for her. My wife and I had reinforced that in several ways, especially if she was scared or in an unsafe situation. However, in her little brain, there was no distinguishing between what she needed me for and the things she wanted me to do.

You may find that your patients and staff have the same problem. They may feel that you should just do whatever they want, not thinking about what they really need or what is best for them. They may also try to draw you into their life drama. Do not make that mistake. It is emotionally exhausting to get caught up in other people's self-inflicted drama.

On the other hand, there are people in your life who actually give you emotional energy. These people are the ones in your life who inspire you and encourage you when things are tough. They can be a spouse, friend, or mentor. I cannot emphasize enough the importance of choosing the right people to spend time with on a regular basis. Do your best to spend regular time with the people who give you energy, as there will always be those around who drain it from you.

Building up your emotional energy requires being very intentional. Things we already discussed, like exercise and sleep, do help. But for those of us who are introverts, having some regularly scheduled alone time is also very important. Solitude can be hard to come by when you are married and have children. One of the things that I do for my wife is to make sure that on the weekends she has a little quiet time to relax while I play with the kids. We love each other and love our children, but sometimes, having a little quiet space is necessary to recharge.

Quiet time is also important for reflection. Too often we are so busy with life that we do not stop to reflect on it. Time for reflection is important for learning from our experiences. Reflection allows us to step back and think clearly. I recommend setting aside even a few minutes every day for this process. I also like to take a half a day or so at the end of every year to reflect. This time allows me to consider what has been working for me and what things I need to do differently. I reflect on things that I am learning. I reflect on the moments spent with my family to solidify those special memories as well.

One way to make that reflection even more powerful is by journaling. There are many different methods for doing this. Your journal can be a simple chronological recording of the major events in your life, or it can be a narrative of all your thoughts, ideas, and dreams. You can buy a special book for journaling or type it out on your computer. There are even apps for journaling now.

Looking back at your journal entries can help you determine if you are learning from your experiences and meeting your goals, or if you still have work to do in a particular area of your life. For example, if there is an idea that you read about in this book today that would be especially helpful to build up your energy reserves, you may make it a goal by writing it down in your journal. In a week or a month from now, you might look back at that journal entry and reflect on how well you have implemented that idea. Were you successful or did you forget about it completely? Journaling allows you to monitor your personal growth over the years.

While quiet time and reflection are beneficial for treating burnout, they must be balanced by social interaction and support. When physicians start to feel burned out, they can start to withdraw from others. Because we spend all day with people, sometimes we just want to be alone after work. This can lead to a vicious cycle of feeling more socially isolated because we are also withdrawing from other people who often want to be of help. Having time for reflection is helpful, but if you start to feel isolated and withdrawn it may be time to seek emotional support.

Without a good balance of physical, mental, and emotional energy it is hard to break through the inertia of burnout and implement the changes needed to reduce stress. Consider where you may be lacking. Do you need to include more activity, rest, or reflection? When your energy accounts are full, you will be better equipped to implement the stress reduction techniques presented in the next chapter.

CHAPTER SEVEN

REDUCING YOUR STRESS LEVEL

Given the multitude of stressors that face physicians, doctors need to find ways to take care of themselves and watch for signs and symptoms of burnout. As we talked about with your energy levels, you simply cannot take care of others if you are not taking care of yourself. We often put our own care last on our long to-do list, which has negative consequences over time.

Let's take a look at some strategies that you can implement to reduce the stressors in your life. These strategies have been effective for many other physicians. Start adding them into your life and take the opportunity to improve your own wellness.

WORK

The first step to reducing stress is to identify the things you can and cannot control at work. The list of frustrations physicians face that stem from our current health care system is quite long, and lack of control at work is high on everyone's list.

As you systematically and thoughtfully list your stressors, highlight those things that you are able to change. If at all possible, avoid wasting your time and energy by dwelling on the things you cannot control. Brooding about the unchangeable leads to feelings of helplessness and worsens the symptoms of burnout. Instead, focus on the changes you can make.

Two major sources of stress for a large percentage of physicians are their schedules and their staffing. The schedule is often one of the biggest challenges. A schedule packed with patients and no flexibility usually leads to running behind all day, and that is stressful for anyone. Work with your office manager and staff to add time between patients or time at the end of the day to allow for the completion of documentation and administrative responsibilities. Add a few minutes to each patient visit or perhaps schedule in a mid-morning or mid-afternoon gap. Some practices schedule a two-hour lunch period with no patient visits to actually have lunch, do paperwork, have team meetings, and regroup for the rest of the workday.

Staff issues are another area of high stress for many practices. If you have staff members who are not doing their job or are doing it ineffectively, then you have two options: you can either work with them to create a plan for improving their job performance or fire them. That may sound harsh, but I speak from experience. Early in my career, I had a staff member who was consistently inconsistent. If she was having a good day, then she was cheerful and efficient in her work. If she was having a bad day, then everyone around her was miserable. With all the leadership and coaching skills, I was learning at the time, I felt certain that I could make her a star employee. I gave her books and paid for classes. We had weekly meetings to talk about her progress.

Things did not go according to plan. Despite some initial success, it became apparent that this person did not have the right attitude and mindset to grow into the type of staff member we needed. After another blow up in the office, I had to admit that it was better for me, as well as the other staff members and patients, to terminate her employment. Physicians spend a lot of their time at work. We need to have a team who will make life easier for us.

While fixing your stressors at work will significantly help to reduce your overall stress, some physicians work in an environment where the process for change is so slow that it also contributes to their stress. When you are burned out you need help fast. The rest of this book is going to focus on strategies you can use that do not require getting approval from an administrator or going to meetings to discuss the need to have meetings about the change you need.

RESTORATIVE ACTIVITIES

One of the best ways to decrease stress is to find restorative activities that you can do on your own. Exercise, sleep, hobbies, and artistic outlets all can reduce your stress and lessen the symptoms of burnout. Some people find massage, acupuncture, or meditation to be quite helpful in stress management as well. All of these have evidence for increasing a sense of wellness and can make a significant difference in how you feel.

It is important to choose something that is truly restorative for you. For example, I find massage is very relaxing and restorative for me, whereas yoga definitely is not. I tried yoga a few times and certainly did not feel restored because my body was not meant to bend into those positions. You, on the other hand, may find it very relaxing. We each have to find activities that restore us.

I find that spending time with family is also restorative. Playing with my children makes me happy. It reminds me why I work hard. The love I get from my family and the joy they bring reduces my stress considerably. French philosopher and essayist Michel de Montaigne wrote, "The greatest joys in life are happy memories, which you can revisit at any moment of time. Therefore, the great business of life is to create as many of them as possible." I certainly try to do that with my family.

Unfortunately, burnout often strains relationships with our spouses and children. Taking our stress out on our family is not the answer, but it happens too frequently. We must be intentional about building good relationships at home.

Developing connections with other physicians is beneficial as well. Relatively few people outside of medicine truly understand what we have gone through to get to this point in our careers. Talking with colleagues can also give you ideas on ways to improve your own practice or grow your career. Conversely, it is also a good idea to make connections outside of medicine to give you perspective on the world outside of the hospital or clinic.

SPIRITUALITY

Spiritual beliefs and religious practices are highly personal and in our current political climate a very sensitive topic. However, multiple research studies show that there are health benefits to practices such as prayer and meditation. Therefore we should not avoid talking about the importance of our spiritual lives when it comes to burnout.

A study of ER physicians in Massachusetts looked at the impact of spirituality on burnout. Burnout was measured using the standard Maslach Burnout Inventory, and negative coping behaviors like smoking, drinking, and drug use were self-reported. Of those doctors who responded, negative behaviors were less likely among those with a religious affinity. This mirrors other research of the general population that shows less depression and lower rates of suicide in those who attend religious services regularly.

LIFE PHILOSOPHY AND ATTITUDE

Many of us do not spend much time thinking about our life philosophy, but doing so can reduce stress. We should have an approach to life that incorporates a positive outlook, identifies and acts on our values and stresses balance between personal and professional life. Not only will such a philosophy make us better people in general, but it will decrease the stress that stems from a life that is lacking in purpose.

Your life philosophy may include giving back to the world around you. Generosity has been shown to have benefits on psychological health. Working on or toward something bigger than yourself gives a life purpose and meaning. Both are often lacking in burned out physicians. It is also important to find meaning in your work. Incorporate that into your life philosophy.

Like most things in life, medicine has its good and bad aspects. But fortunately, our attitude about it is entirely up to us. Attitude is a choice. Psychologist and Holocaust survivor, Viktor Frankl, wrote, "The last of our human freedoms is to choose our attitude in any given circumstances." This makes sense. If we allow our circumstances to dictate our attitude or emotions, then we are giving up control to outside forces. That loss of control worsens burnout.

Fortunately, we can control our attitudes. It is not always easy, but with determined effort it is possible. We must make a conscious effort to catch and correct ourselves whenever we start feeling negative about a situation. It may be a hundred times a day at first, but it will gradually get easier.

Regardless of what problems we face in healthcare, it is important to remember that we are essential to the most important and meaningful aspect of medical practice—the patient encounter. We reap the rewards that come from relieving suffering and restoring health to others. Keeping that perspective can help us better manage the other stressors we face.

In the next chapter, I am going to teach you some of the time-management strategies and skills I have learned over the years from the masters of productivity and success. These experts have over a hundred years combined experience teaching business people and entrepreneurs how to make the most of their time. Now I think it is time for physicians to master these same skills.

CHAPTER EIGHT

TIME MANAGEMENT

Time management courses are full of business people who rarely (if ever) work more than 40-hour weeks. These same courses really should be offered to physicians starting in the first year of medical school. We all could benefit from learning how to manage our most valuable resource.

Nearly every physician I work with faces the same three key challenges when it comes to their time. You likely have the same problems:

- You do not have enough time.
- You do not control the time you have.
- You do not focus on the right tasks at the right time.

Do any of these challenges sound familiar? What if you could find and harness 30 hours of lost time each month? If I can help you do that, then reading this book will be a worthwhile investment of your invaluable time. In this section, my goal is to help you clarify your priorities so that you can take control of your schedule and maximize your productivity.

The single biggest waste of time is to start anything without clear, specific goals. Many physicians waste their most valuable resource by responding and reacting to whatever is going on around them. They spend their careers working to achieve the goals of other people instead of taking the time to become absolutely clear about what it is that they really want for themselves.

By reading this book, you are choosing a better path. As you go through the exercises, you will become clear on your goals and your priorities. You will free up more of your valuable time and have a better work-life balance.

In my coaching program, one of the first activities we do, in conjunction with the Legacy Ladder I wrote about earlier, is highlight which things in that client's life are really crucial. That does not include what someone else thinks is urgent or important. I encourage you to do this same exercise now. Write down the events and activities that are essential to helping you reach the goals that you have crafted with the help of the Legacy Ladder questions.

If one of your goals is to spend more time with your family, write down the dates of your children's birthdays, your anniversary, upcoming graduations, music recitals, vacations, and any other activities do you not want to miss. Then do the same for your career goals. Is there an annual conference that you want to attend? Are there skill building workshops or courses that you need in order to grow professionally?

After you have written down all of the important events in your life, take your calendar and put these things on it. Book that time now so it does not get squeezed out later. Too often, we let the mundane or other people's "emergencies" crowd out the most important things. I understand that there are times when our priorities must take a back seat, but those times should be the rare exception instead of the rule.

After you have blocked out your calendar, the next step is to block out your daily schedule. I use a simple spreadsheet with days of the week across the top and each hour down the left-hand side. Start from the time you wake up. Do you begin with exercise, hygiene, or reading? Make sure to include meals and family time. Commuting and work have to be on there. Remember to include blocks of time for working on your legacy goals as well. Did you include an hour or two a week for learning your needed skills? Do you need a half-hour every day to work on writing your next book? If you do not put your priorities and goals into your schedule they will never get done.

As busy as it may seem, do not get overwhelmed by this new schedule. You do not need to book every minute of every day. In fact, I would recommend leaving a little time in your schedule for spontaneity, a time when you can choose to read a book at home, go for a walk in the park or go out to dinner with friends. The point of creating a block schedule is so that you control your schedule instead of letting others fill it up for you. You can work toward your own goals instead of everyone else's.

Block scheduling is a very effective way to get things done. Carve out 30-minute, 60-minute, or even half-day chunks of time to focus on one project, task, or goal. You will find that you can accomplish so much more by setting aside uninterrupted blocks of time. Turn off all potential distractions during these blocks. Completely focus on one task and only that task. Do not try to multitask. It is the biggest mistake many of us make when it comes to productivity.

What about efficiency? Efficiency and time management go hand in hand. While they are both essential, they are not the same thing. If you are efficient at your work, then you will have more time for the things that are most important to you. On the other hand, you can be very efficient at doing tasks at work, but not manage your free time well. In this case, being efficient may help you get done with work faster, but you are not able to make progress on your personal goals because you do not manage the extra time appropriately. That is why it is so important to hone these two distinct skills of efficiency and time management.

CHAPTER NINE

BECOMING MORE EFFICIENT

Another word for efficiency is productivity. How productive are you with the time that you do have? Are you constantly looking for ways to improve your efficiency so that you can have more free time for yourself and your family? Too often, we blame others for our lack of efficiency.

It may be true that your medical assistant could room patients faster or the hospital staff could turn over the surgical suites faster, but that lag time does not have to be wasted. I do recommend that you encourage your staff to be as efficient as possible and help them see how doing so will benefit them and the patients. However, any dead time can be a time of productivity and you can even start working on tasks that you would have relegated to another time. Tasks that can be squeezed in during that down time may include checking labs, answering emails, or documenting.

I hate when people waste my time. Fortunately, I am learning that I am ultimately in control of my time and that I can decide if that time is really wasted or not. With the power of our current mobile devices, we are no longer limited to reading outdated magazines in the dentist's office or watching TV in the doctor's lounge while we wait. We can update a to-do list, answer messages, research information about complicated patients, and even look up labs or sign off charts. I have even dictated part of this book into an app on my phone while waiting.

That same mobile device, however, can be a major distraction if you let it. One of the biggest enemies of productivity is frequent interruption. It is estimated that the average adult spends three and a half hours a day checking apps, email, and text messages. Those self-imposed interruptions do not include the number of times someone comes into your office and interrupts documentation or other work that you are doing.

Frequent interruptions or working while distracted makes us less productive and more prone to making errors. It breaks the momentum that is created when we get into the flow of a project or task. While it is true that you can start typing or dictating again right away, your efficiency drops significantly compared to when you are "in the zone." Find ways to minimize distractions as much as possible. Close your office door and put up a sign that says you are dictating or charting. Have specific times a day when your staff can bring you all the papers you need to sign. Have them batch questions for the end of the clinic if possible. Turn off the notifications on your phone. Did you know that most smartphones have a do-not-disturb feature? Make use of it regularly, especially when you are trying to get something done that requires lots of focus, or when you want to get done quickly.

DOCUMENTING MORE EFFICIENTLY

One of the biggest areas that most of us want to become more efficient in is documentation. How much of your workdays, or even non-workdays, do you spend charting? For most of us, documentation takes up the majority of our day and dealing with the electronic medical record (EMR) plays a huge role in physician burnout. There are ways to be more efficient with this and take away some of that stress we all deal with regularly.

Would you rather be reading a good book, playing with your kids, or doing really just about anything else, instead of catching up on charts all the time? I certainly would. That is why I have made it a personal goal to learn every shortcut possible in whatever EMR that I am using. The other way to improve efficiency in an EMR is by changing the way you write notes.

The idea of a SOAP note is to be concise, informative, and focus on what other clinicians would need to know when they care for your patient. All you need to include is the pertinent details so that the next person who looks at your note can understand what you found and what you plan to do. I have had some amazing colleagues over my career who wrote impressive notes. They included information such as where the patient lived, what type of house it was, what support system was in place, and if they had any pets. That was just the social history. The problem was that it took an hour to write each note. I felt bad for these physicians because I know they are trying to do their best, but this level of detail was not needed.

SOAP notes do not need to be written to the standards of your college writing professor. It is okay to have fragmented sentences or dangling participles. I have authored multiple books, so I know there is a time and place for quality writing and grammar, but your SOAP note is not it.

Another thing to remember when writing notes is that bullet points are your friend. Think of your note as an outline for the full story. For example, you probably do not have to write out the entire incident about your patient falling off the ladder while trimming the pine trees in his back yard last weekend. Simply put, "Sudden onset 7/10 sharp low back pain after 3-foot fall 3 days ago." Location, severity, quality, and onset are required for documenting a pain complaint. The rest of the story, while it may be interesting to hear, is not necessary to include in the documentation. Avoid the temptation to narrate or over edit your note. It is not an easy change to make, especially at first. The note will not look or read as "pretty," but it still gets the information across and does what it was intended to do.

Another trick to maximize efficiency while documenting is to template everything! Most of you are probably already using templates in your electronic medical records, but are you really maximizing the benefit of these time-saving tools? Most pre-built templates are generic for a reason, to be used by as many doctors as possible regardless of practice or specialty. Make sure to adjust your templates to fit your needs. If you are typing (or even dictating) the same thing more than once a day, you definitely need some kind of template or smart phrase for that piece. I consider myself to be an efficient note writer but I still routinely look for ways to improve my templates over time. It is a continual improvement process.

When I first started my practice, my partner and I had an EMR system that was not user-friendly, so I had a folder of Word documents for everything. This folder included letters to consultants, cover letters for referring doctors, letters for insurance, case managers, attorneys, and anyone else who might need information from me. When I subsequently worked at other facilities, I was able to place those letter templates directly into the EMR and eliminate the need to type in the patient's name, medical record number, date of birth, date of injury, and other information. My efficiency increased dramatically.

One final tip is to consider changing the order of your SOAP note. Many of us scroll down to the Assessment and Plan first anyway, to see what we did at the last visit or what the consultant recommended. It would save time, clicks, and scrolling if you just placed the Assessment and Plan at the top of your note. Even if it saves you no more than 30 seconds per patient, if you are documenting on 20 patients a day, then you will have saved 10 minutes of your time that day. If you multiply that by a week, you will have nearly an hour of your time back (and even more if you see more than 20 patients per day, which many of us do).

So would it be worth changing the order of your note to regain an hour or two every week? Over the course of a year, that is more than 50 hours of your life you will have regained! That is not bad for the few minutes you spent reading these pages.

The electronic medical record is one of the biggest contributors to physician burnout, but unfortunately, it is now a permanent part of our healthcare system. Learning to be as efficient as possible and get the most out of these flawed software systems can go a long way to reducing the stress in your career.

We could spend an entire workshop going over additional time management and efficiency techniques, but for now, I encourage you to start with the ones that I just shared with you. As I mentioned earlier, multitasking distracts our focus. Making one or two successful changes at a time can have a big impact. These few simple changes have freed up countless hours for physicians that I have worked with over the years.

If your schedule is still too full after going through these exercises and making the changes that you have learned, then it is time to consider delegating tasks. While there are many things that must be done in life, they do not all have to be done by you or me. The next section is all about outsourcing as much of your to-do list as you possibly can in order to maximize the efficient use of your time.

CHAPTER TEN

OUTSOURCE EVERYTHING

You can overcome the feelings of overwhelm that many physicians have when they have too much on their plate. How can you do this? You can outsource many of the common tasks on your to-do list. Imagine what your life will look like when you do.

In his book, *The 4-Hour Work Week*, Tim Ferris states, "A lack of time is actually a lack of priorities." That may sound ludicrous in light of all the demands on a physician's time, but it is something we should consider more closely. Many of the things we do on a regular basis probably do not have to be done by us. If we could get better at prioritizing and outsourcing effectively, we could free up a significant amount of time each week.

One of the first steps to becoming a successful outsourcer is to determine what your time is worth. If you, for example, take two weeks off each year, then you will work 50 weeks annually. If you work 50 hours a week, you will be working about 2,500 hours per year. Those who work 60 hours a week, will average about 3,000 hours per year. To determine your hourly wage, divide your annual salary by the number of hours you work each year. For example:

$200,000/2500 \text{ hours} = \$80/\text{hour}$

$400,000/3000 \text{ hours} = \$133/\text{hour}$

This is what your time is worth. Whether you are seeing patients or doing your laundry, your hourly rate would be $80-$133/hour. Would you pay someone else that hourly wage to mow your lawn, do your dishes, or clean your bathrooms? I certainly would not. What other things are you doing now that you could hire someone else to do for a lower hourly rate?

So go ahead and make a list of all the chores you do, and especially those that you have been putting off, like cleaning out the garage. Then write down what it would cost you to have someone else do each task. If you hire the neighbor kid to cut your grass, for instance, he may charge $25 for the hour he takes to do it. If your hourly rate is $133 an hour and his is $25 an hour, why would you cut your own grass? Do you know a college student who needs extra money? Offer her $80 to clean your house every week. If she does it in two hours the hourly rate is $40. Again, you are actually saving money. It may take some time to find the right people to help you with these tasks, but you will be well rewarded when you can spend more quality time with your family and friends, work on a hobby, or do other activities that you have been unable to enjoy because you do not have enough time.

There are two more questions that you should ask yourself when choosing which chores to outsource. First, what time-consuming tasks do you do that are not rewarding? Secondly, what things are you doing that you absolutely hate to do?

If you hate doing a chore, then stop doing it. Life is too short to be burdened with chores we hate. On the other hand, even if you could outsource something at a lower hourly rate, but you really love doing it, then go ahead and continue to do it. My mom loves getting on her riding lawn mower and taking off around the yard where no one can call her or bother her. My wife loves cooking and experimenting in the kitchen, even if it takes up a significant amount of her free time. For them, those activities are relaxing. There is no need for them to give up these activities.

As you start making your own "outsourcing" list, give yourself permission to get creative. Make it a game to see how many tasks you can off-load!

- Grocery shopping

- Lawn care

- Washing the car

- Booking travel for your next CME conference

- Finding the best hotel deals in Hawaii for your upcoming family vacation

- Creating a PowerPoint template for your next presentation

- Finding the perfect weekend activity for your kids within a 30-minute drive of home

- Scanning old journal articles you want to save into electronic format so you can declutter your office

- Making Indian food for dinner one night a week (This is one of the few favorite things we have yet to master making on our own in my house.)

The outsourcing possibilities are almost endless. For those in private practice, with good management and business plans, you can even hire a mid-level or another physician to see your patients for you. You can also bring in a locum tenens physician to cover for you while you go on that vacation of your dreams.

So where do you find all of these mystery helpers? Just ask around. Let people in your neighborhood know that you are looking for someone to take care of your lawn. Tell the people at church that you are looking for someone to clean your house. Call your alma mater and ask if any of the students are interested in part-time personal-assistant work. There are also several web-based companies that provide outsourcing, virtual assistants, or ratings of local service providers. Your only limits are your creativity and your comfort level in giving up certain tasks.

Giving up certain tasks, in fact, that may be the most difficult part of outsourcing. As physicians, we can find it hard to give up control. We are skilled and capable. We are also prone to perfectionistic tendencies, so even if someone does a great job, there is a chance that it will not live up to our high standards. Sometimes it just comes down to the fact that the job would not be done the same way we would do it. But is that really so bad? As long as things get done and get done well, that is what is important.

I have to admit that my personal philosophy has slowly evolved on this issue. Previously, I wanted to do everything myself to ensure it was done exactly the way I expected. I am reaching the point where I would outsource every task and chore in my business and at home if I found the right people to do them. This would leave me with only the few tasks that I really care about doing myself, such as taking care of my kids and sharing what I have learned on my journey with you. Those two things are extremely important to me, and I enjoy them greatly. I would also free up time for doing work that I actually get paid for. If you are seeing patients or catching up on your documentation and billing, you are making money. If you are cleaning your own house or mowing your own lawn then you are losing money and time.

That is why I am here: to help you have a more fulfilling career and lifestyle. I believe you can get rid of burnout. I believe you can take back more of your time. At the end of this book, you will find a link to additional resources on outsourcing if you want to become a master outsourcer.

Up next, I want to address a specific group of physicians who are highly vulnerable to burnout. Being a physician is tough, but being a physician mom adds a whole new layer of stress. I would like to share some resources that can help with the unique stresses that plague women who have to divide their time between their careers and their families.

CHAPTER ELEVEN

GET RID OF MOMMY GUILT

Let's talk about mommy guilt for a minute. Obviously, I am not a mother, but I know several. My wife is a physician mom as is my sister-in-law and several friends from medical school. I have been able to see first-hand the added stress that those two roles can have, especially when they seem to be competing. As I have listened to physician moms, I hear the frustration and guilt they feel for working long hours, being away from their children, and not keeping up their homes like they would like to do.

Many of them have the same concerns, fears, and yes, guilt. One physician mom, whom I will call Jessica, told me, "I work full time and we have no family nearby to help. My physician husband works such long hours that he rarely sees our two toddlers during the week, either. I feel like every single day is just a huge "to do" list of work and there is little enjoyment in our lives." She went on to share that in addition to the stress and fatigue, she feels even more guilty because she thinks that other physician moms are able capable to cook wholesome food for their families, keep the house neat and organized, and also find time to go to the gym. When Jessica does try to spend time outside with her kids, she feels that this is taking time away from getting her chores at home done. She dreads it, knowing that the tasks are piling up with the passing of time.

Her story is hardly unique. I have heard many other physician moms echo the same sentiments. That is why I had to include a specific section in this book for Jessica and other physician moms like her. Being "more resilient" is not really an option when your time and energies are already maxed out. Mindfulness is, at best, only a temporary fix because a physician mom feels the constant pull of the needs of her children, her career, and possibly her spouse. Her work does not end when she comes home from her job. I won't pretend there is an easy button or quick fix that will make all the worry and guilt go away. However, I will reassure you that it can be better.

One of the reasons I enjoy doing workshops so much is that the audience members get to share their feedback. Some of the physician moms in one group shared excellent ideas and practical solutions about what had worked for them. I will tell you what I learned from these moms and from my own home experience, and you can see if these suggestions help you.

The suggestion that I heard most repeated was do not be afraid to get help. The most frequently recommended was, of course, family, followed by babysitters, house cleaners, and lawn care services. Another idea that resonated was finding a meal service that will prepare and deliver meals to your home on a regular schedule.

Outsourcing grocery shopping is also becoming more common. Stores will let you order online or on their app and they put everything in your cart for you to pick up. Better yet, you can have someone else pick it up for you.

Once you get help, it is easier to free up time for taking care of yourself. Many moms talked about how much even a simple exercise routine helped them feel better. It is important to exercise, but do not kill yourself. It has to be something you enjoy or you will not keep it up. If possible, join a gym with a daycare so that you can exercise regularly without worrying about finding childcare every time you want to go.

Clean, healthy eating also came up frequently. Several moms also mentioned the importance of getting enough sleep, even if it meant some chores did not get done. Others listen to podcasts or audiobooks while they commute to nurture their minds or just for relaxation.

Make time in your schedule to do the things that rejuvenate you. For some, this may be just a quiet afternoon to read a book or putter around the house by yourself. Volunteering on a community service project can be invigorating. For others, spending time with family and/or friends is energizing. Most states have parks, zoos, beaches, aquariums, or other attractions for kids within driving distance. Spending time with your spouse or children can enrich the quality of these relationships.

As my wife reminds me, there is no amount of logic or rationalization that will make the mommy guilt go away. Even if I reassure her that the kids are growing up healthy, happy, and well adjusted despite the floor being dirty or laundry unfolded, it does not take away those feelings. But finding ways to lessen her burden—specifically by unloading some of the household chores from her plate—frees her to spend more time interacting with our children instead of cleaning the kitchen. And when she does play now, she does not have to fret that those chores are just piling up for later.

Do not worry about getting it all done. Instead, focus on enjoying your family and your life. You are a physician and a mom. You do not have to choose one or the other.

It may take a while to perfect the skills I am sharing with you, so if you recognize the symptoms of burnout in yourself, ask for help. This applies to all of us. A loving spouse, supportive parents, and caring friends or colleagues can be a great resource for the burned out physician.

There is no shame in reaching out to others in your life who want to support you. We as doctors do not typically like to admit that we are not coping well with our stressors. However, ignoring the signs of burnout can lead to much more serious problems, including depression, impaired relationships, divorce, and, in some severe cases, even suicide. Considering the consequences, it is worth whatever temporary discomfort you might face to seek out the help you need.

One of the most underutilized tools for helping physicians overcome burnout is peer coaching. I specify _peer_ coaching because there are many non-physicians who want to coach physicians. Some of them mean well and truly care about helping, but they do not and cannot understand, however, the full extent of what it is like to be a physician—let alone a burned out physician.

CHAPTER TWELVE

COACHING—THE FASTEST WAY TO SUCCESS

For a large number of physicians, getting back a few hours of their time each week, unloading mundane chores to free up time for more important activities, and strengthening their support system by building better relationships at home can be enough to change the course of their career and their life. For me, those simple things make a world of difference on my mood, my attitude, and my outlook on life. However, there are some doctors who have very unique and very specific situations where these successes alone are not enough to relieve their burnout.

For them, coaching is the best option to tackle the problem. Even if I wrote a book the size of Harrison's Internal Medicine textbook, there would still be unique situations that would not be addressed. I will share some examples of specific individuals.

Robert* is a primary care physician who reached out to me because he was burned out and was contemplating suicide. His biggest source of burnout was not a lack of time, the electronic medical record, or difficulty at home. The problem was that he worked for a rural Federal hospital where he had no control over the patients who were on his schedule. When patients were abusive to him or the staff, he could not fire the patient. There was nowhere else for them to go, so he was required to see them. Even drug-dependent patients who threatened physical harm to him if he did not prescribe what they wanted kept getting put back on his schedule. Discussions with the administration were fruitless.

Claire* had a small solo practice. One day her only nurse became seriously ill and had to go out on FMLA. Claire could not afford to hire a new nurse while she was still paying the first one. She was tempted to just close down her clinic for two weeks while her nurse recovered, but she would still be losing money because she was not working. Even more stressful was deciding whether or not to keep her long-time employee if the medical condition might result in repeated absences for treatment.

Eric* wanted to change jobs. He was tired of working for a large hospital system and wanted to join some colleagues in private practice. Unfortunately, Eric's daughter had been born with a rare disorder that required specialized care and multiple surgeries. He could not afford to have any gap in medical coverage, so he stayed at a job he hated for the daughter he loved. Others in similar situations have told me that they wanted to move but had to stay in certain cities because their loved ones could only be treated at a few facilities nationwide. They felt that their options for getting out of their current situation were limited.

Jennifer* loved her job and had worked there for ten years. A new department chair was recently hired and started making drastic changes, placing more demands on Jennifer and her partners and requiring them to take calls in-house instead of from home. These changes had a dramatic impact on her quality of life, an issue that was more important to her than more money or fewer call days. She had attempted to meet with the new department head to discuss the changes but those meetings kept getting postponed.

* The names have been changed, but the situations are very real.

For individuals like Robert, Claire, Eric and Jennifer, personalized coaching can be the right tool for relieving burnout. There are several unique factors that make coaching ideal for overcoming stressful challenges.

First, coaching is personalized to your specific situation. Not every administrator can be approached the same way. Every job does not have the same opportunities for flexibility or advancement. Not every challenge at home has the same solution. Coaching can identify an individual's strengths and apply them in challenging situations. Coaching can also identify areas for growth and come up with a plan to develop the necessary skills to overcome obstacles.

Each of us has unique strengths, weaknesses, and opportunities. A coach can help you maximize those and reach your full potential. Going through a coaching program can help you become more focused and more effective. You are able to go farther and do it faster than you could on your own. Physicians who try coaching also tend to be more fulfilled in their careers and have a better work-life balance, which leads to less burnout.

A coach can also help you look objectively at a problem. He or she may be better able to see the obstacles and opportunities that you may miss when you are in the midst of the situation. When you are stressed, your emotions start to take over. You can become blinded by fear, frustration, anger, or exhaustion.

Albert Einstein once said, "You cannot solve a problem with the same thinking that got you into that problem." His words apply perfectly to physicians who are experiencing burnout. Your coach can help you step back and see things more clearly from a big-picture view. A coach can help you think outside the box.

Thirdly, your coach is there to serve you. Your coach is not swayed by ulterior motives that an employer, colleague, or even a spouse may have. An employer does not want to have to replace you if you choose to leave. A colleague may fear they will have to do more work if you need a long vacation. A spouse may be concerned about the financial ramifications of cutting back your hours or taking a new job. Your coach is there for you, to help you make the best choices possible to overcome your burnout. He or she has your best interest in mind and wants to see you succeed.

Your coach is your thinking partner. A coach provides unbiased feedback throughout the program in a confidential and non-judgmental manner. Together you can find the best solutions. Your coach is there to help you reach your goals and to hold you accountable along the way.

There are limits to coaching, however. Coaching is not used to diagnose or treat medical issues such as clinical depression, substance abuse or suicidal ideation. An ethical coach will refer these conditions to the proper mental health professionals. It is similar in my medical practice. I am a physiatrist. I treat musculoskeletal conditions. If someone refers an expectant mother to my office I will gladly treat her pregnancy-related back pain. However, I am not going to try to deliver the baby. That would be malpractice. Likewise, a coach can still help you work through challenges and move toward your goals while you are getting treatment for the medical conditions, but they are not a substitute for the mental health specialist.

I have used coaches for several areas of my own life. I have had coaches to help me with marketing, with public speaking, with writing, and even with coaching. I learned more in a much shorter time from having these experts show me the way than I could have on my own. Imagine going through medical school and residency without ever working with an attending physician. How good of a doctor would you be if you just tried to learn it all on your own by reading books or articles online? Those attending physicians, like coaches, taught you many things that you would never learn from the books. They certainly safeguarded you from costly mistakes during the learning process.

The original definition of a coach was "to bring a person from where they are to where they want to be." That may sound simplistic, but it has worked consistently over many generations. I like sports, so I will use a sports analogy. There are many tremendously talented athletes in professional sports. However, the most successful ones are not always the ones who were chosen highest in their respective draft class or those who were considered to have the most potential.

Basketball legend Michael Jordan had immense talent, but he did not win an NBA championship until he had a coach, Phil Jackson, who could unlock his full potential. Another basketball superstar, Kobe Bryant, also demonstrated amazing skill and potential, but like Jordan, he never won a championship until Phil Jackson became the coach of his team. There are many great players who have never won a championship because they did not have the right coach. There are probably many more individuals who had great potential but were never given the opportunity to develop it fully.

This applies to other talents as well. I have heard some amazing singers who aspired to greatness but whose songs will never get played on the radio. I have watched amazing musicians who will never be known outside of their family and friends. I know some incredibly smart doctors who have desired to reach others beyond the confines of their own practice but will never have their own television show or be featured on the cover of a magazine. It is not the lack of talent or potential that is holding them back. It is the lack of the right coach to take them where they want to be.

Regardless of your goals, the right coach can help you reach them faster and with fewer missteps along the way. When you are burned out, you do not want to waste time on theories or ideas that do not work. The trial-and-error method is not the approach you want to take when you need help now.

A coach can help you:

- ✓ Decrease Your Stress Level

- ✓ Maximize Your Career Potential

- ✓ Improve Your Relationships

- ✓ Develop Specific Skills

- ✓ Become A More Effective And Influential Leader

✓ Identify and Overcome Specific Challenges

✓ Make Lasting Change In Your Personal And Professional Life

✓ Become More Efficient With Your Time

✓ Find The Joy And Fulfillment You Had When You Started Medicine

Physician coaching can help alleviate the underlying causes as well as the symptoms of burnout. The negative consequences of not addressing burnout include lost jobs, divorce, substance abuse, and even suicide. And as if these problems were not enough, quality of care and patient satisfaction decrease while the rate of medical errors and malpractice lawsuits increase when physicians practice in a state of burnout. These results speak boldly of the need for physicians to seek appropriate help as soon as symptoms begin. Furthermore, seeking the help of a coach demonstrates professionalism that attempts to provide the best care possible for patients. After all, our mantra is "first do no harm."

I have been asked if I think everyone needs a coach. My answer is this: everyone would benefit from quality peer coaching, but not everyone *needs* it. If after reading this book and taking action on what you learned you are able to have the lifestyle and work-life balance you want, then you may not need a coach for burnout. However, if there are still problem areas that seem to hold you back or goals that you still want to reach, then coaching may be the right answer for you.

Some physicians are so disillusioned by medicine or burnout that they think about quitting medicine altogether. Sadly, some doctors believe this is the only solution to their burnout. Fortunately, there are other options which we will discuss in the next chapter.

SECTION 3:
A Life Without Burnout

CHAPTER THIRTEEN
DO I REALLY NEED TO QUIT?

You can quit at any time. But is quitting medicine and giving up on your career the only solution to your burnout? Medicine can be extremely stressful, and we are practicing in a very tough time for healthcare in general. Before giving up the practice of medicine, however, it is very important to take serious consideration of the costs versus benefits to you and those you care about.

Most of us went into medicine for a good reason. Most of us, at least at the onset of our careers, truly enjoy taking care of our patients. We like being able to help and to heal. Medicine, at its most basic core, is an extremely rewarding profession. Unfortunately, it has been made more challenging by certain policies and protocols that have been formed by politicians, regulators, special interest groups, lawyers, and insurance carriers. Are there exercises that you can do that will enable you to still find the joy in relieving the suffering of your patients?

If you do care about your patients, think about the repercussions to them as well as to your colleagues if you quit medicine. With the current shortage of physicians in this country, those patients will only be foisted on other busy physicians who do not know them as well as you do. If they were your aging parents or children, who would you want to care for them as they get sick? Wouldn't you wish for a physician who has the right training and expertise, especially if they have had a good long-term relationship with your parents or children? If we all quit medicine just because things are tough, people we care about would suffer.

We have worked very hard and sacrificed so much to become physicians. We cannot get back the time, energy, and money we invested in this career. So why not try something less drastic first? Start with some of the things you have already learned in this book, like time management or how to be more efficient. Even if you implement only one small change at a time, the effects will multiply as you continue to find ways to hone your new efficiencies. Become an expert outsourcer. Delegate all the tasks that you do not absolutely need to be doing.

Another essential part of overcoming burnout is to develop good relationships with your staff. Zig Ziglar, a well-known motivational speaker, once said, "You can have everything in life you want if you will just help other people get what they want." If your staff knows that you care about them, they are more willing to work with you to decrease your stress. That may mean that they take on more of your administrative duties, protect you from unnecessary interruptions, or block inappropriate phone calls. Your staff can be some of your greatest allies in battling burnout at the office.

Another very helpful antidote to burnout is to partner with other doctors in your clinic, department, or hospital to come up with ways to lower stress and ease burnout. We know that over half of all physicians experience burnout, so the chances are very high that one of your colleagues is burned out, too. We need to stop acting as though we live and practice on an island,

and we must start working together. That is the only way we are going to improve our healthcare system significantly. In fact, neglecting to work together has resulted in the erosion of our autonomy as physicians. Insurers, regulators, hospitals, and other parties have been able to put more pressure on us as *individual* physicians because we have not worked together to stand up against these large groups and organizations. So reach out to your colleagues, as they can be one of your biggest sources of support if you let them.

Developing a sense of collegiality and community in the physician ranks will also go a long way in negotiations with administrators. Too often the concerns of a lone physician get brushed off. That dynamic changes dramatically when five or ten physicians request to talk with the VP for physician services or the hospital CEO. There is power in numbers. If several of the physicians in your group have the same concerns, take them to administration en mass. I guarantee that it will be more effective.

If you are not getting the results you want in your career or your life, consider hiring a coach. I have already shared the many benefits of coaching as a highly effective tool to help you achieve your goals. Your coach can get you unstuck, or if you still decide to leave medicine your coach can help you make a rational, well-informed decision instead of doing something rash that you might regret later.

Before you give up on your career, also consider taking a vacation to blow off steam and clear your head. Sometimes a brief break is all you need. If you need extended time to recover and consider your options, you should talk to your employer or partners about a taking a sabbatical. While it is not widely advertised, there are some large employers who actually offer sabbaticals to physicians who have been with the company for a certain period of time. It is nice to know that after your time away, you still have a job to come back to if you choose.

One more option that has become more popular recently is locum tenens work. For burned out physicians, this can be a great opportunity to keep practicing medicine without many of the stressors they had to deal with in their previous job. I will share with you my experience in the next chapter.

CHAPTER FOURTEEN

AN ALTERNATIVE WAY TO PRACTICE

Locum tenens has been around for a long time, but it is becoming a more popular career choice for burned out physicians. With this type of work, you do not have the administrative headaches that typically come with running your own practice. You have tremendous flexibility to choose when you want to work and can enjoy a greater work-life balance.

So why do we not hear more about locums as a career option for burned out physicians? I have found that many burnout experts are not familiar enough with this type of work to recommend it. In addition, locums is a different lifestyle, and some physicians are not comfortable with those changes.

I actually had not considered doing locums at first either. When I first started building my speaking and coaching career, I soon realized I would have to either continue to do it on the side or I would have to give up my private practice. It was a tough decision. My practice was doing well, but, on the other hand, I really wanted to help other physicians enjoy their careers more and be able to thrive in their medical practices. When I got married, my wife lived in another state, so I took the opportunity to transition into this new phase of my career.

For two years I was out of clinical medicine, and while there were things about it that I was glad to be done with, there were things that I missed. After all, I went into medicine to help people, and I still found it very rewarding. I found that locums work gave me just the right balance between having my own practice and being a full-time speaker and coach. My first assignment came by chance one day when I was given an opportunity to cover for a friend who wanted to go on vacation. She had an inpatient practice for a large hospital system, but unfortunately, she was the only physiatrist covering the inpatient rehabilitation unit. The person who was supposed to fill in for her learned that he could not get credentialed at the hospital in time for her vacation. They learned about this only two weeks before my friend was scheduled to leave for Hawaii with her family, and she was worried that she would be unable to go with them. I was able to get my credentials for the hospital via a whirlwind process and was there in time for her to make her flight.

That was my first experience as a locum tenens. I was able to take care of patients and avoid all of the administrative headaches that went along with running my own practice. I was paid a fair hourly rate and felt appreciated by not only my friend but also the entire staff who knew she needed a well-earned vacation.

It was not long before I started expanding my locum tenens opportunities. I spent a few months going to cities where I had family, which made my work weeks like a paid vacation with a little work thrown in along the way. I came to appreciate why locum tenens is becoming a popular option for physicians looking for better work-life balance. It is nice to just see patients and not to have to worry about accounts receivable, billing insurance, collections, or managing staff.

My first locums experience did not occur in the typical fashion, however. We were able to complete all the arrangements in a very short amount of time because I already had a license in that state and had previously been credentialed at that hospital. For most assignments, licensing and credentialing typically takes several weeks to several months.

The locum tenens agency will help with getting a state license if you do not have one already. They will work with the facility to get you credentialed. The hardest part for me was locating copies of all my documents, such as USMLE scores, diplomas, residency certificates, board certifications, and case logs for various procedures like EMG and injections.

In most cases, the agency will cover the costs of obtaining and maintaining your licenses, which is helpful once you have more than one or two. They provide malpractice insurance and take care of travel expenses such as lodging, flights, and rental cars. Once they have all of the necessary information from you, they will start actively looking for job assignments that fit your needs.

One thing that is essential to note is that as a locum tenens physician you are an independent contractor. You are not employed by the locums agency or the facilities where you work. This means you will be responsible for your own taxes, health insurance, disability insurance, life insurance, and retirement planning. None of that has to be daunting. Finding a good accountant is an important first step. In my book, *Personal Finance for Physicians,* I outline the basics of what types of insurance most physicians need and which advisors you may want to hire. It can be a good resource as you start out as an independent contractor.

I have found locums to be a great fit for me. I can continue to develop my career as an author, speaker, and coach while still maintaining my clinical skills. When my wife and I had each of our children, I was able to take fewer assignments and devote more time to being the best dad and husband possible. Regardless of what assignments I choose, I am in control of my time and my career path in ways that I never could be if I worked for a large organization. Locum tenens is a novel way to beat burnout. It is a fairly easy solution to implement and works well for many physicians. Locums can be a full-time career or a temporary solution depending on your needs and goals.

If you need a change from your current practice situations, there are alternatives out there for physicians. Locum tenens is one of them, but you may also find other opportunities that fit your needs. Shift-work suits some people's lifestyle better than regular office hours. In residency, a few of my colleagues and I did utilization reviews for workers compensation claims. There are also non-clinical opportunities available in pharmaceuticals, insurance, research, or medical writing to name a few.

I would encourage you not to give up on your medical career completely until you have fully explored all of your options. You worked too hard to get to this point. You owe it to yourself to see if you can make it work. However, there are some people for whom leaving medicine altogether is their best option. I have met a few who went into medicine for the wrong reasons and they never had a passion for it. For them, there was no sense in continuing. Others had health or personal situations that were so bad that they did need to step away indefinitely to address those issues. These instances, fortunately, are rare.

We went into medicine because we were passionate about relieving pain and suffering. We had grand dreams and ideals. We should not walk away just because the passion has waned. My daughter enjoys roasting things over the fire with me. When the fire would eventually die down she would get sad and tell my wife that we could not cook on the fire anymore. I loved watching the excitement in her eyes as I brushed back the ashes to reveal the hot coals beneath. I would add some paper and a few small sticks and the fire would soon be burning hot again. You can do the same with your career. It is possible to rekindle the passion you had when you started. Try some of the options I have suggested here and you may not have to give up on being a doctor.

SECTION 4:
Wrap Up

CHAPTER FIFTEEN

PUTTING IT ALL TOGETHER

Congratulations on getting to the end of this book. It is my hope that reading this has helped you form a plan to overcome stress and create a better work-life balance. I hope that it inspires and motivates you to create your own burnout breakthrough. You invested the time to learn, and I applaud your effort.

But the end of this book is not the end of your journey. There will be circumstances that arise to test your new resolve. Your stressors will still be there tomorrow. Responsibilities will pile up. Good habits are not developed overnight. There will be times when you will need to go back and review your answers to the Legacy Ladder questions. You will need to play the outsourcing game over and over when tasks start piling up again.

The things I teach are simple, but they are rarely easy. We get stuck doing the same things the same way we always did them. Burnout only deepens that rut. It takes work and repeated effort to climb out. But you can climb out. You can overcome burnout, and I believe you will. You have already invested in yourself by taking the first steps with this book.

As author James Allen states, "Everyone wants to improve their circumstances, but most are unwilling to improve themselves, thus they are forever bound." Physicians have access to an immense amount of information, but many never take action.

Sometimes we need someone who knows how to help us reach our goals and hold us accountable along the way. I promised you real, practical solutions to decreasing stress, adding more time to your schedule, and achieving better work-life balance. Now I want you to be accountable.

Post your block schedule where you can see it. Create a family schedule and place it in a central location where your whole family can see it. Create a version for work so staff and colleagues can see when you are available to talk and when you need to be left alone to accomplish what you need to do.

Write out your goals and the answers to your legacy ladder questions neatly on a clean sheet of paper. Tape that paper to your bathroom mirror and read over it while you are brushing your teeth every morning until you have memorized your priorities. You are much more likely to live up to them if you have them ingrained in your brain. Then look at it again every night and ask yourself if you made progress that day toward your goals. Celebrate those wins. Take joy in your successes.

Networking with peers is very helpful to many physicians. We tend to get isolated in our own practices and try to survive on our own. Connecting with colleagues who are in similar situations or who have similar interests can be a good way to cope with stress. My mastermind groups have provided great opportunities for physicians to network, but it is not just my teaching or insight that makes it worthwhile. Participants ask questions, share what they are doing and discuss what has worked for them. I probably learn just as much from them as they do from me during those sessions.

Do not let burnout steal your joy or your sense of accomplishment. If you exercise even ten minutes every day, pat yourself on the back. If you make it home in time for supper every night this week, plan a special dinner for the weekend. You can start making changes in your own life today. You can start small or go all-in at once. Either way, I encourage you to start taking action right now. A life without burnout is so much more rewarding.

If you are struggling to incorporate methods of self-improvement, or just want to achieve your goals faster, I recommend reaching out to a professional coach. A good coach will take you from where you are to where you want to be. The problem with most of us is not a lack of learning or knowledge. It is the lack of implementation. You do not necessarily need somebody just to teach you something new. You need somebody to encourage you to make the changes you already know you should be making—someone to hold you accountable.

What have you got to lose? Or better yet, think of what you have to gain. It is time for all of us to stop talking about the problem of physician burnout and actually do something to cure it.

===

*"If you are willing to change, then
everything else will change for you."*

*"The only way to be certain tomorrow will
be better is to make certain you are growing
today."*

About the Author

Dr. Christopher Burton is a board-certified PM&R physician and author of multiple books, including *Putting Out the Fire: How to Prevent Physician Burnout, Personal Finance for Physicians, Marketing Your Medical Practice,* and more.

He is also an executive director of the John Maxwell team, the world's number one leadership and personal development training and coaching organization. He has served as president for his county medical society, chair of the Florida Medical Association's young physician section, and other leadership positions.

Dr. Burton is an international speaker, presenting on topics such as leadership, communication, strategic planning, goal-setting, time management, and physician burnout. In addition, he provides one-on-one coaching for individuals looking to take their career or organization to the next level.

Contact Dr. Burton for a coaching discovery call or to speak to your organization.

info@christopherburtonmd.com

Bonus Resources

Just a reminder to download your
100% FREE Bonus Resources!

Go to christopherburtonmd.com/BBB

You FREE Bonus Resources include:
3 Ways to Declutter Your Life
Effects of Exercise on Physician Stress
Goal Setting & Legacy Ladder
Outsourcing 101
Outsourcing Vendors
Writing More Efficient Soap Notes

Discover the Keys to Getting Rid of Burnout.

Overcome the things holding you back from
a better work-life balance and
a lifestyle that you really want.

Go to christopherburtonmd.com/BBB

Other Books Available from Christopher Burton, MD:

PERSONAL FINANCE FOR PHYSICIANS

As physicians we are experts in medicine, but we don't typically learn much about business or personal finance in medical school or residency. As a result, many physicians make poor decisions with their money. Many never end up building the kind of net worth they expect.

Personal Finance for Physicians provides a basic overview of topics essential to building and protecting your wealth. These topics include insurance, investing, estate planning, retirement and asset protection. You worked hard to achieve professional success; now it is time to focus on your financial success.

MARKETING YOUR MEDICAL PRACTICE

Medical school doesn't include a class on marketing. So how are you going to get patients? More importantly, how are you going to get the kind of patient you want in your practice? Being a great doctor helps, but it isn't enough to generate a busy practice full of paying patients. The healthcare climate is changing, and physicians need to learn the business of medicine.

Marketing Your Medical Practice covers the basics of marketing your practice. Learn how to develop your own personal brand. No matter what type of practice or specialty, any physician can benefit from *Marketing Your Medical Practice*!

BUYING YOUR FIRST HOME: A GUIDE FOR YOUNG PHYSICIANS

Congratulations! You are ready to buy your first home. Buying a home is an exciting experience, but it can be quite stressful as well. You are about to make a major investment that will impact you and your family for years.

This book will help ensure that buying your home is enjoyable, and teach you how to avoid ending up with a housing nightmare. You will find answers to your most pressing questions—and even answers to questions that you didn't think to ask.

PUTTING OUT THE FIRE: HOW TO PREVENT PHYSICIAN BURNOUT

The majority of physicians will experience symptoms of burnout at some point in their career. This book was written with the goal of helping physicians prevent burnout. This book explores:

❖ The effect of burnout on your professional career, relationships, and personal sense of well-being.

❖ Solutions for reducing stress, increasing energy and building coping strategies.

❖ Novel ways to fight burnout without giving up your medical career.

❖ Methods that leaders and administrators can use to decrease the rate of physician burnout within their institutions.

Special Request

Thank you for reading *Burnout Breakthrough*.

I really appreciate getting feedback from my readers. I would love to hear what you have to say and how this book has helped you.

Please go to:
www.amazon.com/dp/B07KQDP6S6
to leave me a helpful review on Amazon.

Christopher Burton, MD

www.ingramcontent.com/pod-product-compliance
Lightning Source LLC
Chambersburg PA
CBHW071606200326
41519CB00021BB/6883